CAREER AS A PHYSICIAN ASSISTANT

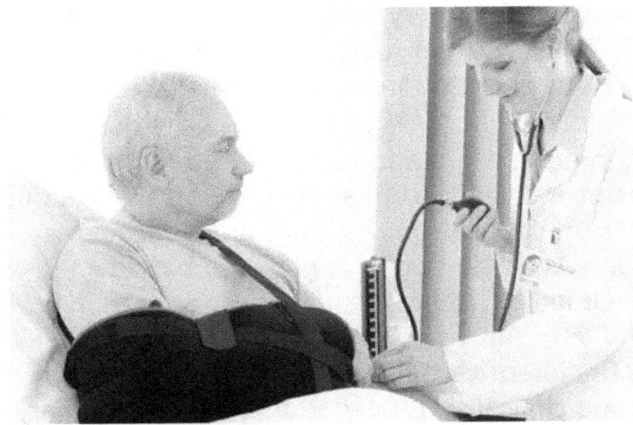

PHYSICIAN ASSISTANT HAS BEEN identified as one of the very best jobs in America. The reasons for the career's appeal are striking:

- Jobs available everywhere

- Relatively fast entry – the post-graduate education averages just 27 months

- Excellent pay starting at around $90,000 with the potential to go much higher

- Flexibility to practice in different specialty areas without additional education

- Job growth that is nearly twice as fast as most other occupations

- Exceptional work/life balance

Physician assistants, commonly called PAs, practice medicine under the supervision of a physician. Their training is very similar to that of physicians, compressed into a shorter period of time. Although they cannot practice independently, they often act as stand-alone providers, performing many of the same duties traditionally reserved for doctors. The actual amount of autonomy they have can vary, but generally they provide diagnostic, preventive and therapeutic services.

Physician assistants are especially important in primary care, where there is an acute shortage of licensed physicians. On any day, a physician assistant in primary care might provide physicals, order and interpret lab tests or x-rays, assist in surgery, diagnose and treat illness, set broken bones, suture lacerations, treat minor burns, prescribe and carry out therapy, and write out prescriptions.

Physician assistant training programs are a fast track into the medical field. Most start with a bachelor's degree, but some programs will admit students with only two years of college courses, granting a bachelor's degree as part of the training. While it is advantageous to have a college major in a subject related to healthcare, especially science, it is not required. In fact, a candidate can enter a PA program with a background in any major. The intensive training programs focus entirely on the medical, scientific, and clinical skills needed to become a primary healthcare provider. Graduates are fully qualified to take certification exams and go to work. No residency is required.

As the healthcare industry continues to struggle with a doctor shortage and a growing patient population, the physician assistant will become increasingly needed. PAs are enjoying progressively greater roles in front-line care as states continually expand the range of services PAs are allowed to perform. It all adds up to fantastic job growth with demand far exceeding the supply of new PAs.

WHAT YOU CAN DO NOW

BECAUSE PHYSICIAN ASSISTANTS have many of the same responsibilities as medical doctors, it is natural to assume that the educational requirements are the same. While physician assistants do spend considerable time in school earning a bachelor's degree, and then a master's degree, the requirements are definitely not the same as for a medical doctor. Physician assistant program graduates, for example, do not have to complete a residency. More importantly, it does not matter what undergraduates choose for a major in college. Physician assistant schools are not looking for any specific major, nor do they look for any particular courses on your high school transcripts.

What you should concentrate on in high school is getting into a good college. Make sure you take all the necessary classes to meet admissions requirements at the colleges you are considering. Your curriculum should provide a solid foundation in math and science. Good communications skills will also be needed, so load up on English, debate, and other classes that can help bolster those skills.

Develop good time management and study skills. You will need them when you get to college. Make it a rule to set aside any distractions and study for a certain amount of time each day. Learn to take good notes in class and review them when you get home. Avoid cramming for tests. Instead, study early, not the night before the test. These simple suggestions might seem obvious, but there are many first year college students who found it easy to get good grades in high school without bothering to learn these skills. Getting into physician assistant school is going to be much harder than getting into college. You will need a very high grade point average, and good study skills are needed to accomplish that.

Make sure a physician assistant career is really what you want. A good way to get a realistic idea of what it is like to be a PA is to job shadow. Shadowing a PA is ideal, but shadowing a doctor can be just as enlightening. Ask your school advisor to help you set this up.

Volunteer in a hospital, clinic, nursing home, hospice, or other healthcare facility. It is a good way to gain insight into the healthcare profession in general, and you might find another profession that you like better, such as nursing, occupational therapy, or radiology. Plus, PA programs will expect that you have some healthcare experience, and volunteer work definitely counts.

HISTORY OF THE CAREER

THIS COUNTRY IS STRUGGLING WITH A doctor shortage. The problem is especially acute in remote and less populated areas, but the challenge of providing healthcare to the entire population exists everywhere.

One obvious solution has been to allow non-physicians to provide basic medical services. There are several noteworthy examples throughout history of this solution in action. In the 17th century, Peter the Great introduced military assistants known as "feldshers' into Russian armies. Feldsher is a German term coined in the 15th century that literally translates to "field shearer." It referred to medieval barber-surgeons who worked as army field surgeons for the German and Swiss Landsknecht (mercenaries) until real military medical services were established by Prussia in the early 18th century.

Although feldshers started out as lower grade army physicians, the concept quickly spread throughout Russia. It became common for feldshers to provide medical services in rural areas and low-income neighborhoods in the cities. Instead of providing emergency surgery on the battlefield, they performed routine checkups, and provided primary care under the supervision of a hospital physician who took on the more serious cases. The system was so successful, it still exists today throughout much of Eastern Europe.

The feldsher system also inspired the famous "barefoot doctors" program in China. After the Cultural Revolution of the 1960s, China trained 1.3 million of these healthcare workers to provide basic medical services to the vast rural populations.

In the US, non-physicians have also long been used to provide healthcare services on the frontiers of the American West, in Native American villages in Alaska, and in underserved rural areas of the South. Long before the profession was established, a highly respected general practitioner in rural North Carolina trained his own "doctor's assistant" to care for patients, even during the doctor's absence. This action was surprisingly well received by the mainstream medical community.

Armed forces, especially in times of war, have always had a particularly difficult time recruiting and training sufficient medical personnel to cover their needs. This reality led to the use of non-physicians to provide emergency care at military bases and on warships in France and England, and in post-revolutionary America. These same military corpsmen were recruited by the US Public Health Service to provide healthcare services in federal prisons.

Following World War II, more and more doctors moved away from general practice, instead specializing in certain areas of medicine. This trend led to a growing shortage of primary care physicians. In 1959, US Surgeon General, Leroy E. Burney, sounded the alarm when he stated that there was a national shortage of medically trained personnel to provide basic medical services to the public. Duke University began a program in 1957 to train nurses to help alleviate the problem, but that program failed and was discontinued less than two years later.

In 1965, Duke University again attempted a training program that would produce qualified healthcare workers capable of providing basic medical services. The program, which was widely heralded in the national press, started with a class of just four ex-Navy corpsmen. The curriculum for this first Physician Assistant (PA) training program was loosely based on the fast-track training of medical doctors during World War II. The program was a complete success, and two years later the profession was officially recognized with the establishment of the American Association of Physician's Assistants (AAPA). In 1970, Kaiser Permanente became the first HMO to employ PAs. To this day, HMOs are a primary employer of physician assistants.

Within four years from the start of Duke's PA program, other academic medical colleges were emulating that prototype. The timing was perfect. The shortage of general practice physicians was becoming critical, compounded by the creation of Medicare and Medicaid, opening access to health services to millions of new patients. Two national commissions, which were formed to address the issue, enthusiastically promoted expansion of all efforts to support the practice of general medicine. By the end of the 1960s, more than 100 programs had been established throughout the country to train physician assistants. The AMA formally endorsed the concept of the "physician's assistant," and began to lay the groundwork for accreditation of programs in order to achieve a common standard of training.

The PA profession became fully established nationwide in the 1980s. By this time, nearly all states had revised statues to allow the PA prescription writing privileges and authorized the delegation of responsibility by the physician to the PA – provided that the tasks were within the scope of the physician's own practice.

Along the way, a new trend emerged. Many PAs started specializing so their employment opportunities would not be limited to general practices. More and more specialization training programs were offered designed to prepare PAs to work for physicians practicing in many specialties. By the end of the decade, the profession was poised for rapid growth.

During the 1990s, the number of accredited PA training programs increased rapidly. Most of the new programs were in smaller colleges affiliated with community hospitals. The number of applicants and admissions soared. Most of the students entered the programs with bachelor's degrees, and graduates were therefore awarded master's degrees.

Because the PA profession has its roots in the military, the first PAs were mostly men. That changed in the 1990s. For the first time, most new PA students were women. Despite the growing number of graduating PAs, there was no shortage of opportunities. In fact, there were still far more job openings than the number of graduates could fill.

At the turn of the 21st century, record numbers of graduating PAs were taking the certification exam. The profession celebrated its 40th anniversary in 2005, as increasing numbers of PAs were appointed to positions in federal agencies, and two were elected to state legislatures. The same year, the US Army and Baylor University created the first doctoral degree program for PAs.

In 2010, President Obama signed the Patient Protection and Affordable Care Act, opening the door for as many as 30 million new patients in search of primary care. More than ever, the country will look to physician assistants to provide those services. Although the 100,000th PA was certified in 2012, many more are needed to join the ranks of this in-demand profession.

WHERE YOU WILL WORK

THERE ARE CURRENTLY ABOUT 90,000 physician assistants employed in the US. Over half are working in doctors' offices. These employers are usually specializing in family medicine, pediatrics, geriatrics, or orthopedics. Another 25 percent work in hospitals. The rest of the civilian PAs are employed by outpatient care centers (typically run by HMOs), public clinics, government health agencies, prisons, outpatient surgical centers, academic medical centers, and private corporations. Basically, wherever there are doctors, there are physician assistants.

It is not unusual for physician assistants to hold two or more jobs, or be self-employed with multiple clients. For example, a PA might work a few days a week at a doctor's office and the other days make the rounds of nursing homes or urgent care clinics.

The profession has its roots in the military, and even today the armed forces depend on PAs to serve as the front line of military medicine. In the Army, physician assistants are known as Medical Specialist Corps officers. These PAs are responsible for all healthcare of soldiers assigned to their unit, as well as their family members. They go where their unit goes, which may be in combat zones during times of conflict. Physician assistants also serve in the Air Force, Navy, and Coast Guard.

The first employer of physician assistants was the Department of Veterans Affairs (then known as the Veterans Administration or VA). Today, the VA is still the largest single employer of physician assistants, employing more than 2,000.

There are also physicians assistants working for the US State Department. Designated as Foreign Service Health Practitioners (FSHP), these PAs are the primary care providers for members of the State Department and their families. Working in this capacity, they may be deployed anywhere in the world where there is a State Department facility.

The work environment for physician assistants is generally indoors in comfortable surroundings. Most work in fixed locations with little opportunity for travel. However, there are a few situations that call for the PA to get out of the office. For example, some physician assistants make house calls or visit nursing homes to treat patients, reporting back to the physician afterward.

Physician assistants must adhere to the hours of the employing or supervising physician. For most, that means working full time with routine hours Monday through Friday. Those who work in hospitals, however, may have to work night shifts or on weekends and holidays. They may also be on call during unscheduled hours. If called, the PA must be ready to come into work with little notice.

THE WORK YOU WILL DO

PHYSICIAN ASSISTANTS, USUALLY known as PAs, practice medicine under the supervision of licensed physicians. They are vital members of the healthcare team, filling the gap between doctors and the nursing staff. Their purpose is to extend and complement the capabilities of the physician. Physician assistants are capable of providing virtually every clinical service except major surgery. They routinely handle uncomplicated health issues such as sprains, strains, hypertension, bronchitis, flu, depression, allergies, asthma, gynecological problems, family planning, and trauma.

The training of the PA is similar to that required for physicians. Therefore, they are qualified to perform routine tasks that would otherwise be performed by doctors. It is estimated that PAs can do about 80 percent of the work a physician does. In general, physician assistants examine patients, diagnose health conditions, and provide treatment. The supervising physician determines specific duties. Once the physician has delegated certain responsibilities, PAs are expected to carry out their duties without further direction. The physician may or may not be present while the PA is at work. In rural and medically underserved areas, for example, a physician may visit a clinic only once or twice a week. In this case, there is little direct supervision. The physician assistant acts as the primary care provider, conferring with the physician only as needed (and as required by law).

A physician assistant working in private practice would typically have a regular schedule of patients to interview, examine, diagnose, and treat. Most of the time, the patients would never see the physician at all. Because the physician assistant is taking care of the routine services, the physician is free to focus on the most difficult and complex cases, while still being available for consultation.

A physician assistant working in a hospital setting is known as a "hospitalist." A hospitalist is responsible for evaluating, treating, and providing continuity of care for patients who have been admitted to the hospital. These are usually patients who are quite ill and require close monitoring. Often they have serious and complex ailments that require extensive nonstop care that is beyond the scope of a nurse's capabilities, but also more time consuming than a physician can provide. Depending on the hospital, PAs may also handle some advanced procedures, like putting in breathing tubes, inserting surgical drainage tubes, starting central IV lines, and treating major emergencies as part of a trauma team. PAs who work in university hospitals split their time between treatment and aiding in research and instruction. In some cases, more experienced PAs will supervise less experienced PAs.

Physician assistants typically perform all preliminary patient interactions. In doing so, the PA lays the groundwork for treatment and saves the physician valuable time. The PA starts with a patient interview, reviewing the medical history and discussing any immediate and long--term health concerns. The patient is then examined and diagnostic tests are ordered if necessary. The PA confers with the supervising physician regarding any observations and recommendations for treatment. The PA is also responsible for keeping the medical histories up to date by recording all services, conditions, and progress.

Diagnosis and treatment are at the heart of the physician assistant's work. Diagnosis starts with the physical examination, but often requires one or more tests to identify or confirm the illness or disease. The PA may administer non-invasive tests, and order X-rays, MRIs, CAT scans, blood tests, or electrocardiograms. When the results of the tests come back, the PA interprets the results to arrive at a diagnosis and determine a course of treatment.

Treatment options that may be performed by a physician assistant include:

- Administering injections and immunizations

- Cleaning, dressing, and suturing wounds and infections

- Setting and casting broken bones

- Prescribing medications

- Ordering or performing therapeutic procedures

- Performing or assisting in minor surgeries

Physician assistants are also involved in educating and counseling patients. This means discussing any chronic conditions, describing what to expect from treatment, and interpreting medical terms for patients and their families. Patients and their families often have questions and it is the PA's responsibility to provide answers. In the case of chronic conditions or situations that may require long-term care, the PA will develop a healthcare management plan specifically for the individual patient. Some physician assistants, particularly those who work in public health clinics, conduct outreach programs where they talk to groups about managing specific diseases and promoting wellness.

Physician assistants who work in private practices often have managerial duties. Depending on the type and size of the practice, the PA may be responsible for:

- Ordering medical and lab supplies and equipment

- Supervising technicians and medical assistants

- Ensuring that the working environment is clean and safe, and in compliance with state regulations

- Managing infectious disease control policies and procedures

- Coordinating technical information

- Developing educational programs

- Maintaining records and certifications

The work of physician assistants depends largely on their specialty and what the supervising physician needs them to do. For example, a physician assistant working in surgery may close incisions and provide care before and after the operation. A physician assistant working in pediatrics may conduct physical exams and give routine vaccinations.

More than half of all physician assistants practice primary care medicine, which means being the first contact for people with health related problems. PAs in primary care usually work in a doctor's office or a health clinic. Primary care is an umbrella term that includes the practice of family medicine, internal medicine, pediatrics, and obstetrics and gynecology. Like the physicians they serve, PAs can follow many career paths. There are dozens of different specialties a physician assistant can choose. Some of the most popular choices are:

Surgery

Surgical physician assistants work under the supervision of a surgeon, conducting preoperative tests and physical exams. They also act as first assistant during surgeries, even before other surgeons. Surgical PAs can do some surgical procedures on their own, such as putting in chest tubes or cutting and draining abscesses. They also may be tasked with monitoring a patient's recovery after surgery and continuing to provide follow-up care. Surgical subspecialties, such as thoracic, orthopedic, and plastic surgery, are becoming increasingly popular.

Emergency Medicine

Physician assistants who crave excitement often find their calling in the emergency room. Working in the ER, a PA will see patients with all types of medical conditions, ranging from a mild case of the flu to life-threatening injuries. Most emergency PAs deal with patients who are generally stable, and have simple and straightforward needs. The most common procedures are suturing and wound care, splinting and wrapping sprains and strains, refilling medications, and treating colds, infections, rashes, and minor burns.

Orthopedics

PAs specializing in orthopedics work alongside doctors, assisting with surgeries on broken bones. They also work independently, resetting dislocated bones, making and removing casts, and performing live imaging procedures like fluoroscopy.

Psychiatry

Mental health work involves interviewing patients who are in mental distress, suicidal, depressed, or suffering from dementia. Physician assistants who are certified in this specialty are able to prescribe medications and give injections of long-term medications to patients with ongoing mental illnesses.

Dermatology

A dermatology physician assistant may evaluate and treat a wide variety of skin disorders and diseases. Some also perform cosmetic procedures.

The supervising dermatologist determines exactly what a dermatology PA will do. For example, duties may be limited to dealing with skin rashes, acne, or the removal of skin tags and moles. The dermatologist may also have the PA assist with more serious surgical procedures, such as removing skin cancers.

Urgent Care

Urgent care clinics, which may be independent businesses or affiliated with a hospital, bridge the gap between private doctor offices and hospital emergency rooms. PAs in these clinics provide medical care for injuries and ailments that are not life threatening, but still require treatment. Urgent care PAs are often the only provider patients will see. Supervising physicians are often not onsite, but the PAs on staff still work under their direction.

PHYSICIAN ASSISTANTS TELL THEIR OWN STORIES

I Work in a Hospital Emergency Department

"I started my career when this career field was still very new. Even though it was a new profession at the time, opportunities were abundant. It was great being a pioneer while being able to go anywhere I wanted with my career. Since then I have worked in a range of settings from surgical suites to community clinics.

For the last five years I have worked in the emergency department. It is nothing like what you see on TV or in the movies. Patients come here for all sorts of reasons, whether they need critical care or not. I never know what I'm going to see. It could be a sore throat or a heart attack. My job is to provide basic care services and pass on more acute cases to the resident physicians.

There is a licensed physician in the department 24 hours a day, and at least one PA on duty at the same time. The day is broken into two 12-hour shifts. I might see anywhere from 25 to 40 patients during a shift. Typically, I order labs and x-rays, and interpret the results. Sometimes I order the appropriate treatment. Other times, I will refer a patient to a physician who may be a specialist. I rarely see a patient more than once because most don't need additional care. Patients who do need additional care are admitted to the appropriate department, where another PA will take over the responsibilities for basic care.

Many people have asked me why I didn't become a physician. After all, I do much of the same work and have very similar responsibilities. Why not get paid more as a medical doctor? Being a PA has advantages. It gives me time to spend with my family. Most doctors don't share that luxury. I also like having the option to move on to different things. I'm not tied down to one particular job situation.

My advice to new PAs is to be humble and continue to learn everything you can. Always remember that you are there to help and comfort people, not dazzle them with your medical knowledge. This field is not something that you should take lightly. Seeing the smile on a person's face when you've taken their pain away is a reward worth more than any paycheck."

I Am a Rural Family Practice PA

"I was always interested in medicine, but wasn't sure how I would get involved until I job shadowed a physician assistant. I had already shadowed two physicians, and the difference between the careers was striking. For the PA, the focus was on medicine rather than financial matters, dealing with insurance reimbursements, and other management issues. I wanted to treat patients, and being a PA would allow me to do that. I never considered practicing in a rural setting, but during the rural medicine rotation in school, I fell in love with the idea. I knew it would be a challenge, but I was up for an adventure and have never regretted my decision.

Unlike some other PA specialties, the scope of practice is quite extensive in rural family medicine. There aren't enough healthcare providers to go around, and no one thinks about limiting my responsibilities to routine tasks. I see patients of all ages with every health need imaginable. It is not unusual to take care of several generations of a single family. For many of my patients, I am their doctor, their only doctor. Most have never seen my supervising physician and probably never will. They come to me for all their healthcare needs – pregnancy tests, diabetes management, broken arms, strep throats, burns – you name it.

The work of a PA is a unique balance of dependence and autonomy. I can't practice independently, yet I get to see most of my patients on my own. The doctor doesn't have to be looking over my shoulder to make sure patients are being properly cared for. At the same time, I am not alone. If I am unsure and I need guidance, my doctor is always reachable. In case of an emergency, the doctor is less than an hour away.

Being a PA also offers the opportunity to live a balanced life. Doctors sacrifice a lot, especially in their personal lives. They work long hours, have a huge amount of responsibility, and have to spend much of their time dealing with things that have little to do with practicing medicine.

As a PA, I enjoy the perfect balance. I get to help people be healthy, while I live a full life outside of work. My advice to future PAs is to always strive to maintain that work/life balance. It will help you stay grounded and avoid burnout. You will be a happier person, which translates into better patient care."

PERSONAL QUALIFICATIONS

BECOMING A PHYSICIAN ASSISTANT IS a good career choice for people who are interested in medicine and want to be involved in patient care. A passion for medicine and a desire to help people are certainly a good start, but there are other strengths, skills and personal traits needed to be successful in the field. Some of the most important traits are described below.

Effective communications skills

Physician assistants must make the complicated understandable. It takes exceptional communications skills to explain medical concepts to patients, especially considering most of them will have limited medical science literacy. Not only will you see patients every day who have trouble reading and understanding health information, for many,

English is their secondary language. Interacting with other medical professionals on your team or at other hospitals or clinics can also be a challenge.

Emotional stability

Do you handle stress well? As a physician assistant, you will often find yourself in stressful situations. This is particularly true for those working in surgery or emergency medicine, but at any time you may confront a situation that calls for immediate attention and action. It is important to remain steady in order to make the right decisions and provide quality care.

Sometimes both patients and their family members become upset over their situations. They may feel scared, confused, angry, or overwhelmed. Physician assistants must respond to all types of situations calmly without letting their own feelings get in the way.

Detail oriented

Physician assistants must be focused, observant, and detail oriented. This is easy in a quiet classroom, but quite challenging on the job in the flurry of daily activity. Small details can sometimes make all the difference when it comes to a patient's treatment. For example, missing the fact that a patient has a medication allergy could result in serious complications or even death. PAs are also responsible for charting information about the patient's care, and the information needs to be complete and accurate for future reference.

Compassion

Do you have a genuine desire to help people? Most physician assistants are drawn to the profession because they truly care about people. This job is not just about treating and diagnosing patients. It requires giving your all and doing everything you can to help your patients feel better. Being caring and compassionate are a big part of what you do.

Problem-solving skills

Medicine is complex. Patient symptoms do not always follow the textbook definitions. Treatments that work well on some patients, do not have the right effect on others. Sometimes it requires investigative work to make a correct diagnosis or come up with the best treatment plan. Physician assistants need to use considerable problem-solving skills to solve complicated medical issues. That may mean ruling out what does not work through some trial and error, and being willing to try different approaches to find the solution.

Adaptability

Every patient is different and physician assistants never know what the situation with the next one will be. You could be doing one thing one minute and, at the moment you step into the next examining room, you need to shift your focus to something completely different. That is the nature of the job. The work is unpredictable, and situations change quickly. A physician assistant needs to be able to shift gears quickly.

ATTRACTIVE FEATURES

THERE ARE MANY GOOD REASONS TO pursue a career as a physician assistant. The most commonly cited are excellent pay and bountiful opportunities. They do not earn as much as doctors, but the median annual income for PAs is about $90,000. Add an in-demand specialty and move to the right location, and that number can top $125,000 not including benefits. With that kind of income potential, you might think the field is flooded with job seekers, but it seems no matter how many new physician assistants are added, the need far surpasses the supply. In fact, according to government labor statistics, there will be a huge growth of almost 40 percent in job openings for this profession over the next 10 years. Consider the razor-thin unemployment rate of not more than one percent among PAs, and you have one of the most stable careers imaginable.

Big paychecks and unprecedented job growth are just the beginning. Successful PAs say this is deeply satisfying work that is never boring. A day in the life of a physician assistant is anything but routine. There is an element of unpredictability that keeps things interesting. As a PA, you never know who is in the next examining room. It could be a child with a cold, a college athlete with a torn ligament, or an Alzheimer patient who has burned himself. Whatever the case, the PA must be ready to switch gears quickly and provide the appropriate care.

Physician assistants never have to feel stuck in a particular job setting.

PAs have more choices than many other healthcare professionals. There is a variety of work settings to choose from – rural clinics, prestigious teaching hospitals, emergency rooms, oversees military medic stations, and acute care clinics. Work schedules are usually steady at 35 to 40 hours a week, but if the 9 to 5 routine is not for you, there are options. Many PAs choose to work part time to raise young families, take more classes, or pursue other interests. Some even work per diem, taking on temporary assignments when and if they choose to in order to have more freedom.

Physician assistants can also switch fields. Most PAs practice in primary care and family medicine, but there are dozens of areas where a PA can specialize. Physician assistants have the ability to change focal points throughout their career, from orthopedics to surgery to pediatrics and more.

Physician assistants in primary care practice are immune from the soaring costs of malpractice insurance. A primary care doctor's premiums can run upwards of $20,000 a year, while a PA may pay less than $600 per year. Certain higher-risk specialties do cost more for both the doctor and the assistant, but the PA still has the advantage of lower premiums.

The working conditions are good, too. Physician assistants work in clean, well-equipped doctors' offices, hospitals, clinics, and other healthcare facilities.

Most doctors love their work, but hate the paperwork and battling insurance companies. Physician's assistants get to skip all that. Instead, they can spend their time doing what they were trained to do – conducting physical exams, ordering lab tests, prescribing medications, and treating patients.

Unlike doctors, people thinking about becoming a physician assistant can take their time making the final choice to pursue this career. Aspiring doctors must follow a pre-med program in college, but physician assistant programs generally will accept any bachelor's degree. That makes it ideal for any college graduate – even one who has been preparing for a completely different career – to change direction and train to become a physician assistant in a few short years.

UNATTRACTIVE ASPECTS

ALTHOUGH WORKING CONDITIONS are good, the work itself can be both physically and emotionally demanding. Physician assistants spend much of their time on their feet, making rounds and evaluating patients. Those who work in hospitals have the heaviest workout, moving from patient to patient. Those who work in operating rooms often stand in one place for hours at a time without a break. The work can be stressful, too, but the tougher the case, the more rewarding it can be.

For most PAs, the working hours are ideal. They work five days a week and make it home for dinner every night. However, those who work in hospitals do not usually have it so easy. Their work schedules may include weekends, evenings, and holidays. Shift assignments can change without notice, ruining plans to spend quality time with the family. Plus, you are often on call, so days off are not really totally free time. A leisurely afternoon on the golf course can suddenly be interrupted by an emergency call followed by a trip back to the hospital.

Physician assistants enjoy considerable flexibility, but they are not in complete control of their daily routines. They are assistants, which means they still have to work under the supervision of a doctor. Even though they do many of the same procedures as doctors, they are not the ultimate decision-makers on patient treatment.

The schooling needed for this career can be intense. It is certainly not as tough as medical school (not to mention the three or more years of exhausting residency doctors must complete after graduation), but it is not easy. PA training programs are designed along the medical school format, but squeezed into two or three years.

After completing the courses required in a PA program, graduates still have to pass a national certification exam. All that and they still are not done. PAs are required to take ongoing medical education classes (at least 100 hours of classroom time every two years), and they must retake the certification test every six years to maintain their national certification.

Getting into a PA program is not easy. The competition can be tough, especially since most applicants are already nurses, EMTs, or paramedics who already have a healthcare background.

EDUCATION AND TRAINING

PHYSICIAN ASSISTANTS TYPICALLY need a master's degree from an accredited PA program. Earning that degree usually takes at least two years of full-time postgraduate study. While admissions requirements vary from program to program, most programs require two to four years of undergraduate courses with a focus in science. The admissions process is tough and competitive. The most typical applicants are nurses, emergency medical technicians (EMTs), and paramedics with more than four years of healthcare experience.

Physician assistant programs include both classroom and laboratory instruction. Courses may include subjects such as pathology, human anatomy, behavioral science, physiology, pharmacology, hematology, microbiology, immunology, genetics, and medical ethics. The programs also include hundreds of hours of clinical training under the supervision of a physician. Students participate in clinical rotations that typically include family medicine, internal medicine, surgery, geriatrics, obstetrics and gynecology, emergency medicine, and pediatrics. There are usually opportunities for additional elective rotations for those interested in particular areas of practice.

Because of the uniquely close working relationships with physicians, physician assistant training is specifically designed to complement physician training. PA students share many classes and rotations in clinical medicine with medical students who are working towards an MD degree.

There are currently 190 accredited PA programs in the United States, represented by the Physician Assistant Education Association (PAEA). Most programs are graduate programs that lead to master's degrees in Physician Assistant Studies (MPAS), Health Science (MHS), or Medical Science (MMSc). All require a bachelor's degree and scores from two tests: the GRE (Graduate Record Examination and MCAT (Medical College Admission Test.

Licenses, Certifications, and Registrations

All states and the District of Columbia require physician assistants to be licensed. After completing the coursework required in a PA program, graduates have to pass a national certification exam. The Physician

Assistant National Certifying Examination (PANCE) is administered by the National Commission on Certification of Physician Assistants (NCCPA). After passing this exam, a physician assistant can use the credential Physician Assistant-Certified (PA-C). Certified physician assistants may also add these initials after their names: APA-C (Army flight surgeon assistant), RPA or RPA-C. The C indicates Certified and the R indicates Registered. The R designation is unique to a few states, mainly in the Northeast. Most PAs use PA-C.

Certification does not mean all education is completed. PAs are required to take ongoing medical education classes. A PA must log 100 Continuing Medical Education (CME) hours in the classroom every two years. Plus, certification only lasts 10 years. At that time, a PA must successfully complete the Physician Assistant National Recertifying Exam to maintain national certification.

Advanced Specialties

Like medical doctors, physician assistants can choose to pursue a specialty. This requires additional education. There are currently 49 programs in various specialties. The most popular are surgery, emergency medicine (trauma critical care), oncology, neurology, and psychiatry.

PA postgraduate programs are clinical training programs that focus exclusively on learning the specialty field being pursued. There is little, if any, classroom instruction involved. Nearly all training is provided through hands-on, supervised clinical experience. To enter one of these programs, a physician assistant must be a graduate of an accredited program and be certified by the NCCPA.

EARNINGS

PHYSICIAN ASSISTANTS ENJOY EXCELLENT earnings. The median annual income for these professionals is over $90,000. Few PAs earn less than $65,000 a year. Those who do are typically working in poor, rural areas that simply do not have the resources to offer more. There are physician assistants who earn twice that much. Those whose salaries are in the top 10 percent earn more than $125,000 a year. Actual income for an individual will vary depending on the specialty, practice setting, geographical location, and years of experience.

Of the top five settings in which most physician assistants are employed, hospitals offer the highest pay. PAs working full time in hospitals – whether the facility is run by the government, university, or private entity – earn about $95,000. Earnings for PAs in outpatient care centers is about the same at $94,000. Although physicians employ the largest number of PAs, a doctor's office is not likely to offer the highest pay. However, it is still a respectable income of just over $90,000. The lowest pay goes to those who work in education institutions and for various government agencies. Their income is just under $90,000.

The best way to boost income is to pursue a high-paying specialty. There are many specialties a physician assistant can choose from, but the top 10 based solely on average salaries are listed below. Note every specialty on the list offers pay that is well above the national average.

Radiology Physician Assistant
$150,000

Mental Health Physician Assistant
$126,000

Emergency Department Physician Assistant
$116,000

Surgical Physician Assistant
$110,000

Urgent Care/ Walk-In Clinic Physician Assistant
$104,000

Hospitalist Physician Assistant
$102,000

Nursing Home/ Long-Term Care Physician Assistant
$101,000

Internal Medicine Physician Assistant
$99,000

Occupational Health Physician Assistant
$98,000

Dermatology Physician Assistant
$98,000

Most physician assistants receive good benefits, with typical packages including health and life insurance, paid vacations, sick leave, and retirement pay. It is also common for employers to cover the cost of liability insurance, registration fees with the Drug Enforcement Administration, state licensing fees, and credentialing fees.

OPPORTUNITIES

UP AND COMING PHYSICIAN ASSISTANTS have a bright future ahead of them. This career ranks number 2 on CNN's Money Magazine list of best jobs in America, and Forbes has listed it in the top spot as the best master's degree for jobs.

After predicting that the demand for physician assistants will increase by almost 40 percent over the next decade, the government labor department named it one of the fastest growing professions in the US. It will have an astounding rate of growth – nearly twice the normal job growth for the majority of other occupations. The number of new graduates entering the employment pool is not keeping up either. The result is virtually zero unemployment in this occupation. The job outlook for physician assistants could not be better.

Historically, the need for physician assistants has been greatest in rural and medically underserved areas. While this continues to be true, the demand now is across the board in every area in the country. There are a number of factors behind this new reality, including the following:

- Chronic diseases

- Aging population

- The Affordable Care Act

- Physician shortage

- Budgetary pressures

The most common chronic diseases and conditions are heart disease, stroke, cancer, diabetes, obesity, and arthritis. A report issued by the CDC (Center for Disease Control) stated that about half of all adults (about 117 million Americans) have one or more chronic health conditions. One in four adults has two or more chronic conditions. The increased prevalence of chronic diseases and conditions in the US is a driving force behind the need for more PAs who are needed to provide preventive care and treat those who are already afflicted.

It is an unpleasant fact that health tends to deteriorate with age, and the US has a rapidly aging population. This is partly due to a large Baby Boom generation, but also, ironically, better healthcare has increased longevity. In the year 2000, about 12 percent of the population was over 65. By 2030, that number is expected to be almost 20 percent. More importantly, the number of people over 85 – the group most likely to need healthcare services – is projected to increase by 350 percent!

When President Obama signed the Affordable Care Act in 2010, the stage was set for rapidly increased demand for healthcare services. It is estimated that as many as 30 million people will have access to primary care services for the first time as a direct result of federal health insurance reform. There are not nearly enough doctors to meet this demand. Physicians assistants will be needed to fill the gap.

Like the rest of the world, a physician shortage in the US has become more serious in recent years. According to the AAMC (Association of American Medical Colleges), the US will face a shortage of more than 131,600 physicians by 2025. Half of those empty positions will be in primary care and the rest will be spread throughout various specialties. More physician assistants will be needed to take on the role of primary care provider.

Around the world, rising healthcare costs are claiming a larger share of national budgets. One way to address cost containment is to use more physician assistants, who can perform many of the same services as doctors. It is expected that PAs will have a larger role in giving routine care because they are more cost effective than physicians.

The number of positions available to physician assistants is also expected to expand as states allow PAs to do more procedures, and insurance companies agree to cover those physician assistant services.

GETTING STARTED

THE JOB MARKET FOR PHYSICIAN assistants is hot! Most new PAs are able to line up permanent positions even before graduation, either through their school's career center or through connections made during internships or volunteer work. Finding a job is easy. The goal should be to find the right job, not just the first job that is offered. The key is to start early – at least six months before graduation. That allows for plenty of time to determine what you want to do, where you want to live, and what the choices are. Also, keep in mind that the hiring process at many hospitals takes more than three months.

Start by signing up for one or more recruiter listserv. There are many recruiters on Twitter that post hundreds of jobs every week. Ask around to find out which ones are the best and follow them. Post your profile on LinkedIn. Make sure it is complete and looks professional. Then start making connections.

Check the online job boards. There are numerous websites that feature jobs specifically for healthcare professionals. Some are sponsored by professional associations, while others are stand-alone job sites. Either way, these sites make it easy to search for PA jobs in specified locations and specialties. Be sure to post your résumé for prospective employers to see. The best online job board for PAs can be found on the Joblink page of the American Academy of Physician Assistants website. At any given time, there are about 1,000 jobs listed.

Network, network, network. This should start well before you begin applying for jobs. As a PA student, you will come into contact with dozens of PAs, MDs, professors, and other healthcare professionals. You can cultivate good professional connections while interning, volunteering, and shadowing.

You never know who might be the key to your finding the job of your dreams. Share your interests with family members and friends. They might know someone in the medical community who is in a position to hire a PA, either now or in the future.

If you want to work for a hospital, skip the career sites and go directly to the hospital websites. Hospital jobs are commonly posted on the hospital site and nowhere else. Call and visit the department you want to work in directly. Do not submit an application online through human resources. There is a good chance your application will end up in the slush pile. Calling a PA or department manager directly could lead to an invitation to come in for an interview that otherwise never would have happened.

Not sure what kind of practice you want to work for? Sign up at an employment agency that specializes in part-time and/or temporary healthcare jobs. These are also known as locum tenens agencies. There are even some online agencies that specialize in locum tenens physician assistants. Working temporary assignments is the perfect way to experience many different specialties and settings – even in different parts of the country.

Once you have an offer that appeals to you, it is time to negotiate. Never say yes to the first offer. You will never know if you could have gotten a few extra thousand dollars tacked onto your salary or some more in continuing medical education money, if you do not ask. The worst they can say is no. They are not going to take back their offer if you negotiate in a tactful manner. In fact, most employers expect it and consider it the professional thing to do.

ASSOCIATIONS

■ **American Academy of Physician Assistants Information Center**
http://www.aapa.org

■ **National Commission on Certification of Physician Assistants**
http://www.nccpa.net

■ **The Physician Assistant Education Association (PAEA)**
http://www.paeaonline.org

■ **Society of Army Physician Assistants**
http://www.sapa.org

■ **Association of Family Practice Physician Assistants**
http://www.afppa.org

■ **Association of Postgraduate Physician Assistant Programs**
http://www.appap.org

■ **Naval Association of Physician Assistants (NAPA)**
http://www.napasite.net

■ **Veterans Affairs Physician Assistant Association**
http://www.vapaa.org

■ **American Academy of Surgical Physician Assistants**
http://www.aaspa.com

PERIODICAL

■ **Journal of the American Academy of Physician Assistants (JAAPA)**
http://www.jaapa.com

WEBSITES

■ **LocumTenens.com**
http://www.locumtenens.com/physician-assistant-jobs

■ **The PA Life**
http://www.thepalife.com

www.ingramcontent.com/pod-product-compliance
Lightning Source LLC
Chambersburg PA
CBHW070800180526
45168CB00004B/1695

* 9 7 8 1 5 1 1 5 0 0 5 9 3 *